Carnivore Diet For Depression

A 14-Day Step-by-Step Guide To Managing Depression with Curated Recipes and a Meal Plan

copyright © 2020 Brandon Gilta

All rights reserved No part of this book may be reproduced, or stored in a retrieval system, or transmitted in any form or by any means, electronic, mechanical, photocopying, recording, or otherwise, without express written permission of the publisher.

Disclaimer

By reading this disclaimer, you are accepting the terms of the disclaimer in full. If you disagree with this disclaimer, please do not read the guide.

All of the content within this guide is provided for informational and educational purposes only, and should not be accepted as independent medical or other professional advice. The author is not a doctor, physician, nurse, mental health provider, or registered nutritionist/dietician. Therefore, using and reading this guide does not establish any form of a physician-patient relationship.

Always consult with a physician or another qualified health provider with any issues or questions you might have regarding any sort of medical condition. Do not ever disregard any qualified professional medical advice or delay seeking that advice because of anything you have read in this guide. The information in this guide is not intended to be any sort of medical advice and should not be used in lieu of any medical advice by a licensed and qualified medical professional.

The information in this guide has been compiled from a variety of known sources. However, the author cannot attest to or guarantee the accuracy of each source and thus should not be held liable for any errors or omissions.

You acknowledge that the publisher of this guide will not be held liable for any loss or damage of any kind incurred as a result of this guide or the reliance on any information provided within this guide. You acknowledge and agree that you assume all risk and responsibility for any action you undertake in response to the information in this guide.

Using this guide does not guarantee any particular result (e.g., weight loss or a cure). By reading this guide, you acknowledge that there are no guarantees to any specific outcome or results you can expect.

All product names, diet plans, or names used in this guide are for identification purposes only and are the property of their respective owners. The use of these names does not imply endorsement. All other trademarks cited herein are the property of their respective owners.

Where applicable, this guide is not intended to be a substitute for the original work of this diet plan and is, at most, a supplement to the original work for this diet plan and never a direct substitute. This guide is a personal expression of the facts of that diet plan.

Where applicable, persons shown in the cover images are stock photography models and the publisher has obtained the rights to use the images through license agreements with third-party stock image companies.

Table of Contents

Introduction   7
What Is the Carnivore Diet?   10
    Carnivore vs. Keto   11
    Warnings   14
Carnivore Diet for Treating Depression   17
    Why a Carnivore Diet might help treat depression   17
    What do experts or studies reveal about the Carnivore Diet for treating depression?   19
Other Benefits of the Carnivore Diet   21
    The Benefits of the Carnivore Diet   21
    More Benefits Specifically for Women   22
14-Day Guide to Stick to the Carnivore Diet Plan   30
    Coping with these changes   31
    Easing into the Carnivore Diet   32
    Sample 14-Day Guide   34
    Foods included in the Carnivore Diet Plan   37
    Foods to Avoid in a Carnivore Diet   40
Sample 7-Day Carnivore Diet Meal Plan   41
Sample Recipes   44
    Bacon Chicken Bites   45
    Baked Chicken Breast   47
    Beef and Liver Burger   49
    Healthy Beef Brisket   51
    Beef Heart   53
    Blackened Shrimp   54
    Chicken Enchilada   56
    Crispy Chicken Thighs   57
    Crockpot Shredded Chicken   58
    Grilled Chicken Kebabs   60

Grilled Flank Steak	61
Italian Burgers	62
Lamb Chops	64
Lime Coconut Skirt Steak	66
Moroccan Kouah	68
Pork Tenderloin	70
Prosciutto-Roast Beef Tenderloin	72
Roasted Chicken	74
Salmon Filet with Garlic and Pepper	76
Salmon Wrapped in Bacon	77
Steaks with Olive Oil	79
Conclusion	**81**
FAQ	**83**
References and Helpful Links	**85**

Introduction

In recent years, the conversation around mental health has taken a significant shift, moving towards a more holistic understanding of what contributes to our overall well-being. Among the myriad of approaches and strategies to manage mental health issues, diet plays a pivotal role, often acting as a cornerstone for building a stable foundation for mental wellness.

The Carnivore Diet, known for weight loss and reducing inflammation, is now studied for potential effects on mental health, especially depression. This guide explores how adopting it could help manage depression. Consider how your diet impacts not just physical but mental health. With depression affecting many, effective strategies are vital. The Carnivore Diet, usually linked to physical health, shows promise for managing depression.

The idea may seem unusual at first - a diet of solely animal products to address a complex issue like depression. Yet, many reports and new research indicate this diet's potential impact on mental health. This guide explores the Carnivore Diet's core principles and discusses how reducing plant-based foods significantly could enhance mood and cognitive function.

Envision a life where managing depression involves integrating a dietary approach alongside traditional methods like medication or therapy. The Carnivore Diet, with its focus on meat, fish, and animal products, offers an intriguing possibility for those seeking balance and well-being through their dietary choices. This guide is your companion in exploring the science, personal success stories, and practical advice for adopting this dietary approach with a focus on mental health benefits.

In this guide, we will talk about the following;
- The basics of the Carnivore Diet and how the diet benefits its followers in general
- How the Carnivore Diet can treat depression
- Examples of people who were able to manage depressive symptoms through the Carnivore Diet
- Other benefits of the Carnivore diet and how it can help you achieve overall health
- What you'll experience during the first few weeks on the diet
- Steps on how to ease into the diet
- The foods to consume and to avoid

- A 14-day guide on what to eat and what to buy on the Carnivore Diet
- A comprehensive 7-day meal plan with recipes

Whether you're skeptical, curious, or already on the path to exploring dietary interventions for mental health, this guide serves as a comprehensive resource for understanding the Carnivore Diet's role in managing depression. Without promising a cure-all solution, it aims to equip you with knowledge and insights to make informed decisions about your health and well-being.

What Is the Carnivore Diet?

The fundamental principle of the Carnivore Diet revolves around consuming exclusively animal-derived foods while avoiding any plant-based items. This diet primarily focuses on obtaining energy through fats and proteins, with an almost negligible intake of carbohydrates. Foods that are not included in the Carnivore Diet encompass all plant-originated items such as fruits, vegetables, nuts, grains, seeds, and legumes.

The foundational components of the Carnivore Diet consist of a variety of animal products, including but not limited to organ meats, the fattier cuts of red meat, eggs, fish, and poultry, as well as bone broth, lard, tallow, and bone marrow. Additionally, individuals adhering to this diet may opt for high-fat, low-lactose dairy options such as heavy cream, butter, and aged cheeses.

Individuals adhering to a stringent version of the Carnivore Diet avoid consuming tea and coffee, as these beverages are derived from plants. Moreover, strict practitioners also limit their use of seasonings, most of which originate from plants, with salt and pepper being notable exceptions. Nonetheless, it is common for many following the diet to still incorporate various seasonings into their meals.

Carnivore vs. Keto

The Ketogenic Diet (Keto) is a diet focused on meat consumption. While both diets stress protein and fat, Keto allows limited carb intake. It aims to shift metabolism from glucose to ketones for energy. Low carb, high fat intake offers an alternative energy source for tissues, promoting healthy weight loss.

The Carnivore diet is often considered an upgraded version of the Keto diet as it focuses on higher protein and fat intake while excluding starchy vegetables. This diet allows only animal foods, without strict rules on timing or portions. Simply eat until full and satisfied.

Both diets permit fat and protein while restricting carbohydrates, but the Carnivore diet approach seems to be more extreme and restrictive. Thus, it is safe to say that the Keto diet is far more flexible and practical than the Carnivore diet.

Other major differences between these two diet meal plans are as follows:

Carb Intake

While those on the Carnivore Diet aim for zero-carb consumption, the Keto Diet allows the consumption of 5 to 10% carb calories. Those on the Keto Diet eat the animal-based foods consumed by those on the Carnivore Diet, yet Keto followers can eat low-carb plant-based foods.

Food Cravings

Following a Carnivore Diet means you will be increasing your fat and protein intake and eliminating all carbs. You will also be drinking lots of water throughout the diet program. Those on a keto diet may experience mild-moderate cravings, but people on a carnivore diet can have intense, starvation-like cravings. Some dieters give in to their cravings which makes them go back to Day 1 of the diet program.

Meal Frequencies

Depending on how many calories you want to consume in one day, you can have 5-7 meals per day in a keto diet program. This can help reduce food cravings and eliminate feelings of hunger. But if you're on a carnivore diet program, you can only have 3-4 meals a day. Although you can increase your daily eating frequency, your mind and body won't tolerate it.

Macronutrient Ratio

- The Ketogenic Diet commonly uses a 60/30/10 ratio - 60% fats, 30% protein, and 10% carbs. This diet allows some plant foods and spices.
- The Carnivore Diet, on the other hand, focuses on meat without a specific macronutrient ratio. It mainly involves consuming fat and protein, with minimal to zero carbs.

Need for Dietary Supplements

It's a fact that Keto and Carnivore diets limit fruits and veggies, key sources of vitamins and minerals. On a Ketogenic Diet, you can get nutrients from keto-friendly options. With the Carnivore Diet, you may need Vitamin C supplements due to the strict animal-based focus.

Precautions

While you get protein and other vital nutrients from consuming Carnivore diet-approved foods, you may also be missing out on other essential nutrients that can be derived only from plant sources.

When you're on a meat-only diet, you may not be getting the following essential nutrients:

- *Vitamin C*. Important for the stimulation of collagen synthesis. This powerful antioxidant also boosts

immune function and helps reduce the risk of chronic illnesses.
- ***Vitamin K2***. The fat-soluble vitamin reduces blood vessels' calcification. Vitamin K2 also helps reduce the risk of cardiovascular diseases and improve bone and dental health.
- ***Vitamin E***. It prevents lipoproteins and lipids' oxidation. This fat-soluble vitamin and antioxidant also help protect your cells from damage.
- ***Calcium***. The mineral is needed for muscle contraction, nerve transmission, and healthy bones.

The Carnivore Diet may also be deficient in health-supporting phytonutrients. The plant-derived phytonutrients help protect against environmental threats, like attacks from disease and insects. Some of the common phytonutrients are beta-carotene, curcumin, resveratrol, and quercetin.

Warnings

Note that the Carnivore Diet is not suitable for all. The following group of individuals should never try following the Carnivore diet:

Pregnant Women

Due to the lack of scientific research and increased risk of nutrient deficiencies, pregnant women should never follow a Carnivore diet. This may also be bad for the developing baby.

Elderly

The majority of the elderly population has compromised immunity. People 60 years old and above are also more susceptible to different forms of diseases caused by nutrient deficiency. Following a Carnivore Diet can disrupt the normal functioning of the elderly which may result in weakened immunity.

People with Chronic Kidney Disease (CKD)

The Carnivore Diet, high in protein, can be harmful for those with kidney issues like Chronic Kidney Disease (CKD). Excessive protein can build up in the blood, causing nausea, vomiting, weakness, and appetite loss. It may elevate kidney filtration rate, worsening conditions and potentially leading to fatal outcomes.

People who have limited access to organic meat

Not all people can afford to buy organic, grass-fed meat. If you think you don't have the financial resources for high-quality meat, the Carnivore Diet may not be for you.

Those in good health

Healthy individuals should avoid attempting an all-meat diet as it may compromise their well-being. Scientific evidence supporting the Carnivore Diet's benefits is lacking. Consult a doctor or dietitian before starting this diet to ensure it's suitable for you. Understanding the precautions and potential health benefits is crucial.

Carnivore Diet for Treating Depression

Most of us feel sad at times due to loss or struggles. Sadness is temporary and manageable, while depression persists, causing feelings of helplessness and worthlessness. If you show these signs, it could be clinical depression, a treatable condition.

Look out for symptoms like persistent morning sadness, constant fatigue, lack of productivity, difficulty concentrating, loss of interest in activities, excessive daytime sleep, and feelings of worthlessness. Recognizing depression may take time, but loved ones may notice changes. Timely intervention for depression is crucial to prevent harm.

Why a Carnivore Diet might help treat depression

The Carnivore Diet's exclusive focus on consuming animal products while excluding plant-based foods has sparked interest in its potential benefits in addressing depression. This interest is based on anecdotal reports and preliminary research indicating a connection between diet and mental well-being.

Key reasons the Carnivore Diet may be beneficial for treating depression include:

- *Gut-Brain Axis*: The diet promotes gut health, which is crucial for mood regulation and emotional well-being due to the direct communication pathway between the gastrointestinal tract and the brain.
- *Essential Nutrients*: It provides a rich source of nutrients essential for brain health, including B vitamins (notably B12), omega-3 fatty acids, iron, and zinc, which are linked to lower depression rates.
- *Inflammation Reduction*: By focusing on low-inflammatory foods, the diet may reduce chronic inflammation, a condition associated with the onset of depression, thus potentially alleviating depressive symptoms.
- *Blood Sugar Stability*: Eliminating sugar and refined carbs helps maintain stable blood sugar levels, avoiding mood swings and energy dips that can worsen depression.
- *Simplified Diet Choices*: The diet simplifies eating decisions, potentially reducing the daily stress and anxiety associated with meal planning and food selection, indirectly benefiting mental health.

While further research is necessary to fully understand the relationship between the Carnivore Diet and depression treatment, these key factors suggest that this dietary approach could offer a novel avenue for individuals seeking alternative methods to manage depression.

What do experts or studies reveal about the Carnivore Diet for treating depression?

The Carnivore Diet is being explored for treating depression but faces skepticism in the medical community. Health concerns include constipation, colon inflammation, and scurvy from a meat-only diet. While some claim its effectiveness, experts stress ongoing research for conclusive results.

Key points regarding the Carnivore Diet and depression include:

- *Skepticism from Experts*: Health professionals express concerns over potential negative effects associated with excessive meat consumption, emphasizing the need for more research to validate the diet's effectiveness in treating depression.
- *Ketogenic Diet Connection*: Some experts highlight the mood-enhancing benefits of ketogenic diets, which increase ketone levels in the body, potentially improving brain function and reducing depression symptoms.

- *Animal Studies*: Research, including a 2017 review on mice, suggests that ketogenic diets can decrease anxious and depressive behaviors. These diets have also demonstrated anti-inflammatory properties that support brain health.
- *Inflammation Suppression*: Studies by researchers at the University of California, San Francisco, have explored how ketogenic diets may suppress inflammation, offering insights into possible therapies for diabetes, stroke, and brain trauma.
- *Therapeutic Potential*: Beyond mental health, the ketogenic diet has been utilized as a therapeutic intervention for various conditions, including epilepsy in children, due to its anti-inflammatory effects.
- *Anecdotal Success*: High-profile individuals like Jordan Peterson and his daughter Mikhaila Peterson have publicly shared their positive experiences with the Carnivore Diet in treating depression and other health issues, despite acknowledging the lack of scientific backing and offering personal consultations rather than medical advice.

These highlights underscore the ongoing debate and investigation into the Carnivore Diet's role in mental health, pointing to both anecdotal successes and the need for further scientific exploration to fully understand its impacts and mechanisms.

Other Benefits of the Carnivore Diet

The Carnivore Diet is trending and the number of people following it is increasing. People on the diet have also reported various benefits from following the all-meat diet.

The Benefits of the Carnivore Diet

Some of the reported benefits of the Carnivore Diet include the following:

Restricts Calories, Promotes Weight Loss, and Mimics Fasting

The protein-rich Carnivore Diet is filling. Eating this way unintentionally restricts calories, leading to reduced IGF-1, insulin, and growth hormone levels. Calorie restriction effectively reduces inflammation and eases autoimmune disease symptoms, also promoting weight loss.

Low-Residue Diet

A low-residue diet limits high-fiber foods such as nuts, whole grains, fruits, seeds, and vegetables. It's often prescribed for people with irritable bowel disease to alleviate symptoms like bloating, diarrhea, abdominal pain, and gas. The Carnivore Diet, rich in meat, which is easily absorbed in the gastrointestinal tract, can help soothe the gut for both women and men.

Alters the Gut Microbiota

The consumption of an all-meat diet alters rapidly the gut microbiota. The Carnivore Diet significantly increases bile-tolerant organisms and decreases the level of microbes that metabolize various plant fibers. Changes in the gut microbiota could significantly impact health.

Has the Same Benefits as the Keto Diet

Some of the benefits of the Carnivore Diet are due to the body being in a ketosis state, which is the main concept behind the Ketogenic Diet. The Keto Diet can help with various medical conditions like Alzheimer's disease and Parkinson's disease.

More Benefits Specifically for Women

Women, especially, get to experience a few extra benefits. When you consume foods that are acceptable to the Carnivore Diet, you get to feel more energized and focused.

Other benefits of the Carnivore Diet for women include:

Skin Food for Anti-Aging and Better Skin

Carbs and sugar can harm the skin by triggering inflammation, leading to issues like rashes, acne, and premature skin aging. Sugar molecules attaching to protein fibers in cells cause glycation, limiting collagen's ability to rebuild skin structure.

This process accelerates collagen breakdown and reduces hyaluronic acid, the skin's natural moisturizer. Experts equate glycation with skin problems from sun exposure and smoking, amplifying their effects.

Opt for the Carnivore Diet for better, younger-looking skin by boosting anti-aging foods and avoiding those that age skin quickly. This diet eliminates carbs and sugar intake, reducing skin inflammation symptoms. With the Carnivore Diet, achieve glowing, youthful, clear skin sooner.

- *Carnosine and Zinc.* The Carnivore Diet comprised of the consumption of fish, beef, and chicken naturally contains added nutrients like carnosine and zinc. Carnosine helps protect you against advanced aging while zinc helps in wound healing.
- *Omega-3.* When you eat fish, you are benefiting from an anti-inflammatory boost with Omega-3 fatty acids. When you're on the Carnivore Diet, you also reduce the consumption of Omega-6 fatty acids, which can lead to inflammation.

- ***Retinol***. The Carnivore Diet is beneficial when you eat foods like liver and egg yolks, which are rich in retinol. Retinol is beneficial for the skin and can help in dealing with wrinkles and acne.
- ***Bone Broth Benefits***. Bone broth is essential for the Carnivore Diet. When you consume bone broth as part of a healthy diet, you can experience cellulite reduction, a delay in the appearance of wrinkles, glowing skin, and stronger teeth.

According to Body Ecology author, Donna Gates, bone broth can help decrease cellulite's appearance, and it can make your skin more smooth-looking and supple. Bone broth has collagen and several nutrients that help build beautiful and strong skin.

Improves Brain function

There are claims that the Carnivore Diet can help improve cognitive function and mental clarity for all individuals, women included. According to this study, children who undergo an all-meat diet are more likely to maintain excellent cognitive function in their adult years. In another Korean study, it is found that children and teenagers who consumed more meat and poultry gained excellent scores on some cognitive tests.

A study in underdeveloped parts of China explored the link between an all-meat diet and dementia. Findings indicated a lower cognitive decline in older individuals linked to two dietary patterns: one focusing on fruits, veggies, and mushrooms, and the other on soy and meat.

There are carnivore dieters who reported that this diet may help increase mental focus, boost energy, and improve reasoning. This may be related to carbohydrate restriction as an essential part of the diet.

But this may also be related to fat-adaptation and utilizing ketones for energy. Studies show that ketones contain abundant neuroprotective properties and the human brain prefers utilizing fats for energy than carbs.

May help prevent autoimmunity

It is estimated that 6.7 million or almost 79% of persons with autoimmune diseases are women. An autoimmune disease is a condition in which your immune system is destroying the healthy cells of your body.

According to these studies, zinc, which is abundant in meat, can increase Tregs (regulatory T-cells) that prevent an autoimmune response. Vitamin B6, which is abundant in meat, can improve the symptoms of people suffering from lupus, an autoimmune disease.

May help improve symptoms of female reproductive disorders

The increased levels of Vitamins B and D, cysteine, and omega-3 fatty acids in a balanced Carnivore Diet may help improve endometriosis symptoms, according to these studies. Vitamin D in fish may also help symptoms of PCOS (Polycystic Ovary Syndrome) such as pain, acne, and irregular periods. The Myo-inositol, which is present in different meats, can also be of great help.

In a study of 57 women, it was found that a high-protein, low-carb diet can aid in glucose metabolism, effective weight loss, and managing PCOS symptoms. It is important however to note that these studies are not supported by concrete scientific pieces of evidence and clinical trials.

Weight Management

Very low-carb or no-carb diets like Carnivore Diet and Keto Diet can be a good strategy for managing weight and/or promoting weight loss. Based on one approach, low-carb diets decrease insulin production which in turn, prevents fat accumulation and promotes weight loss.

Another reason for this weight loss thing is the absence of sugar in any carnivore diet meal. Any form of sugar may promote weight gain and can cause metabolic diseases such as diabetes. Lastly, protein increases satiety which makes you feel full and satisfied. This will help women dieters consume fewer calories and prevent overeating.

May help decrease inflammation

Women who suffer from anti-inflammatory diseases such as arthritis, asthma, and diverticulitis may benefit from an all-meat diet. Based on research, a well-designed Carnivore Diet can induce ketosis which has a variety of health benefits. In this study of overweight adults, a very low-carb Keto Diet was found to be effective in reducing oxidative stress and inflammation.

This may also be true in a Carnivore Diet. Oily fish such as sardines and salmon are rich in omega-3 fatty acids, a known anti-inflammatory agent. Incorporating this in your meal plan may help relieve pain and inflammation caused by anti-inflammatory diseases.

May help boost libido

Obese and overweight people are more likely to suffer from sexual problems. According to American researcher and psychologist Martin Banks, Ph.D., sexual problems in obese individuals are more common compared with normal-weight individuals. Obese women who follow a Carnivore Diet have more chances of losing weight than those who do not.

Thus, they are also more likely to have improved sexual function. According to a diet enthusiast, one of the important benefits of the all-meat diet is it increases your energy levels throughout the day. This may improve your sex life and prevent sexual disorders like impotence and lack of libido.

Meat and fish, key in the Carnivore diet, are high in arginine, promoting sexual health for all. Iron and zinc in meat help health and prevent diseases. The diet addresses chronic conditions affecting libido by rebalancing hormones like testosterone and estrogen, potentially enhancing sex drive.

May be effective in treating digestive issues

Many people believe fiber is essential for healthier digestion. But this popular belief is opposed by those who follow a carnivore diet, with scientific evidence to back it up. A 2016 study found that reducing the fiber intake of a person with chronic constipation may help improve symptoms such as gas, strain, and bloating. In another study, it was found that a zero-fiber diet (like the Carnivore Diet), may help reverse constipation and can treat constipation symptoms.

May be effective in treating digestive issues

Many people believe fiber is essential for healthier digestion. But this popular belief is opposed by those who follow a carnivore diet, with scientific evidence to back it up. A 2016 study found that reducing the fiber intake of a person with chronic constipation may help improve symptoms such as gas, strain, and bloating. In another study, it was found that a zero-fiber diet (like the Carnivore Diet), may help reverse constipation and can treat constipation symptoms.

Convenience

Compared to other popular diets such as Mediterranean, Alkaline, Atkin's, etc., the Carnivore Diet is much simpler and way too convenient. After all, this diet is just all about eating meat and meat products and drinking water.

Again, there are no concrete pieces of evidence or scientific research that will back up the above-stated benefits. If you are still more than willing to give it a try, follow this 14-day guide for a successful carnivore journey.

14-Day Guide to Stick to the Carnivore Diet Plan

The Carnivore Diet is relatively easy to follow. You don't have to think about the number of calories you take each day. The most important thing about following the diet is being aware of the foods you eat. If you're on a diet, always be mindful of what and what not to eat.

During the adaptation period, you may be experiencing symptoms related to the Carnivore Diet, especially withdrawal-related symptoms. These symptoms are your body's natural response to carbohydrate restriction and elimination of addictive chemicals and agents.

Some of these symptoms include headache, brain fog, sore throat, chills, dizziness, digestive issues, irritability, jaw soreness, muscle soreness, poor focus, and diarrhea. You may also notice or suffer from cramping, insomnia, rapid heart rate, and nocturia or night sweats.

Coping with these changes

In the carnivore Diet program, the first 2 weeks are considered the hardest. Your body starts to adjust to an abrupt change in your usual eating patterns. The physiological and psychological symptoms stated above may give you a hard time while taking the first part of the challenge. The worst that can happen is you'll experience a breakdown that may lead to giving–up.

To help you deal with these changes, here are a few things to follow:

1. **Take a series of blood tests**

   Before starting the Carnivore Diet, get baseline blood tests. These help you and your doctor understand your health status and metabolic needs. Monitoring your health through blood tests is crucial to assess if the Carnivore Diet is suitable for you. After 2 months, repeat tests to evaluate the diet's impact on your body.

2. **Learn to manage your appetite**

   Expect that your appetite will fluctuate during the adaptation period of the diet program. There will be days when you want to eat more than usual and days when you won't even dare think about eating. You need to strictly follow the guidelines in your program and stick to them until your body gets used to this new way of eating.

3. **Don't dare quit**

    During the first week of the diet program, you may feel unwell with flu-like symptoms like fever, headache, and muscle weakness. This is normal as your body adjusts to using fats for energy. Though challenging, don't quit. If severe symptoms like extreme dehydration or breathing issues occur, seek medical help. For practical tips on starting the Carnivore diet, keep reading below.

Easing into the Carnivore Diet

An average of 14 days is enough for you and your body to adjust to your new lifestyle. Here are some tricks to help you adapt to the Carnivore Diet. You need to eat more meat, take electrolytes, hydrate, and take supplements to deal with gastrointestinal problems, sweat, and sleep.

More meat

As you begin the diet, you experience a lot of hunger. Dive in and eat more meat. Make sure to eat lean cuts of meat.

Electrolytes

Since you lose a lot of water on the diet, you also lose vital electrolytes like potassium, sodium, magnesium, and chloride. To compensate for the lack of sodium, add more salt to flavor your meals.

To compensate for the loss of electrolytes, you can consume bone broth or take oral supplements. There are supplements for potassium and magnesium that are available in the market. Ask your doctor about it.

Water

Water is important for hydration, just don't drink water excessively.

Supplements

Supplements are needed to deal with gastrointestinal issues as you ease through the diet. When you abruptly eliminate certain food groups, you may start to experience issues like GI stress and diarrhea. Some supplements include lipase, ox bile, and Betaine HCL. Ask your doctor before taking these supplements.

Sweat more

Exercise is vital as it helps you to sweat more, which is a natural form of detox. As you are giving your body the nutrition it needs, you also get to expel toxins. Help your body detox through sweating and exercise.

Sleep

During the adaptation period, insomnia can be common. To counter this, you must try to sleep before 11. You should also not eat too close to your sleeping time.

Sample 14-Day Guide

Plan for one week. It will help you save time and prevent any hassle in the long run. Throughout the 14 days, you are adjusting to the diet, you'll find that you only need to take care of your shopping list, where to buy the ingredients for your meals, and what you eat three times a day.

Days 1 to 7

What to buy for the week?

- beefsteak
- pork belly
- salmon
- ground beef
- lamb chops
- pork chop
- chicken
- chuck roast

Sample Breakfast, Lunch, and Dinner

Day 1

- Grilled salmon
- Beef steak
- Roasted fatty fish

Day 2

- Eggs and ground beef

- Roasted pork belly
- Ground beef

Day 3

- Salmon and eggs
- Roasted lamb chops
- Seared beef steak

Day 4

- Chicken
- Roasted fatty fish with butter or
- Tallow, slow-cooked beef steak

Day 5

- Grilled chicken
- Ground beef
- Chuck roast

Day 6

- Lamb chops
- Roasted pork chop
- Roasted fatty fish with butter or tallow

Day 7

- Herbed lamb chops
- Beef steak
- Beef steak

Days 8 to 14

What to buy for the week?

- beefsteak
- cod
- beef liver
- ground beef
- bone marrow
- chuck roast
- ribs
- salmon
- chicken

Sample Breakfast, Lunch, and Dinner

Day 8

- Salmon and eggs
- Beefsteak and a side of beef liver

Day 9

- Grilled chicken
- Ground beef
- Bone marrow

Day 10

- Grilled chicken and eggs
- Ground beef and beef live
- Roasted cod with butter or tallow

Day 11
- Salmon
- Beefsteak
- Ribs with tallow

Day 12
- Beefsteak
- Bone marrow
- Chuck roast

Day 13
- Chicken fried steak
- Beef steak
- Ground beef

Day 14
- Cod with eggs
- Slow-cooked beef steak

Foods included in the Carnivore Diet Plan

You can buy food online or at your neighborhood stores. These stores include your local butcher's shop or grocery store, the farmers' market, and big-name stores like Costco, Whole Foods, and Trader Joe's.

You can sparingly consume dairy products like ghee, butter, and cheese. Some of the Carnivore diet-approved foods include:

- ***Red meat*** – pork, beef, lamb, birds, wild game
- ***Organ meat*** – kidneys, liver, heart, tongue, brain
- ***White meat*** – turkey, chicken, seafood, fish, sushi, sashimi
- ***Eggs*** – goose eggs, chicken eggs, duck eggs
- ***Animal fat*** – tallow, bone marrow

Note: When buying meats, especially beef, choose organic, grass-fed meats as they are considered healthier choices.

Why grass-fed meats?

Grass-fed meats simply mean the animals are fed 100% grass for their entire life. The truth is the term grass-fed isn't just a marketing strategy used by butchers or meat sellers to get lots of money. Research shows that grass-fed meats are healthier than conventional meats.

Though you can't easily ignore the fact that these meat choices are slightly expensive, the beneficial effects these may bring are worth every penny.

The following are the benefits of grass-fed meat/beef:

Fewer calories

Compared to conventional meats, grass-fed meats contain significantly low amounts of fat which is considered a smart choice. This means you can eat more meat daily with less guilt.

1. ***More omega-3 fatty acids***

   These healthy fats are abundant in grass-fed meats, especially beef. Omega 3 fatty acids can help reduce inflammation, lower triglyceride levels, and lower blood pressure.

2. ***Low amounts of saturated fats***

   Grass-fed beef contains lower amounts of saturated fats compared to regular beef. This can help reduce the risk of cardiovascular diseases such as hypertension, abnormal heart rhythm, and heart attack.

3. ***May fight against cancer***

   A grass-fed beef/meat has conjugated linoleic acid (CLA) which can help disarm cancer-producing cells in the body. If proven effective, this can be the next breakthrough in cancer treatment.

4. ***Healthier beef/meat option***

   When you consume grass-fed meats, your chances of getting sick are extremely low. This is because you are eating antibiotic-free and hormone-free meat choices.

5. *Safe for the environment*

Raising cattle in the field is far less harmful to our environment than backyard raising. The amount of emitted green gas in the grassland is lower than that in the backyard. You are helping Mother Earth when you consume grass-fed beef.

Foods to Avoid in a Carnivore Diet

Following a Carnivore diet may instruct you to avoid the following foods:

- Fruit: blackberries, strawberries, banana
- Vegetables: potatoes, broccoli, cauliflower
- Nuts: almonds, macadamia, peanuts
- Grains: flour, cereals, bread, etc.
- improve ice cream, protein bars, chocolate, etc.

Sample 7-Day Carnivore Diet Meal Plan

Following the Carnivore Diet involves the elimination of plant-based foods from your diet. You may only eat fish, meat, and eggs. Moreover, you can consume low-lactose dairy products sparingly.

Foods that you can eat on the diet include chicken, beef, lamb, pork, organ meats, turkey, sardines, salmon, white fish, and limited quantities of hard cheese and heavy cream. Bone marrow, lard, and butter are also allowed.

The diet's proponents argue that consuming fatty meat cuts reaches your daily energy requirements. The diet encourages you to drink bone broth and water but does not allow you to drink plant-based beverages like coffee and tea.

The Carnivore Diet does not have any specific guidelines as to serving sizes, calorie intake, or how many snacks or meals to eat daily. Many of the diet's proponents suggest the consumption of food when you want to.

However, since you're just starting, you can refer to the sample seven-day meal plan to establish a structure. When you have been on the diet for a while, you can eat as often as you desire.

Below is a sample seven-day meal plan to highlight the Carnivore Diet's simplicity.

Day 1

Breakfast: Bacon Chicken Bites

Lunch: Beef and Liver Burger

Dinner: Blackened Shrimp

Day 2

Breakfast: Baked Chicken Breast

Lunch: Beef Brisket

Dinner: Crispy Chicken Thighs

Day 3

Breakfast: Chicken Enchilada

Lunch: Beef Heart

Dinner: Crockpot Shredded Chicken

Day 4

Breakfast: Grilled Chicken Kebabs

Lunch: Grilled Flank Steak

Dinner: Lamb Chops

Day 5

Breakfast: Italian Burgers

Lunch: Lime Coconut Skirt Steak

Dinner: Moroccan Korah

Day 6

Breakfast: Salmon Filet with Lemon and Garlic

Lunch: Prosciutto-Roast Beef Tenderloin

Dinner: Pork Tenderloin

Day 7

Breakfast: Salmon Wrapped in Bacon

Lunch: Roasted Chicken

Dinner: Steaks with Olive Oil

Sample Recipes

Here are some of the easy-to-prepare Carnivore diet recipes that you and your loved ones can enjoy.

Bacon Chicken Bites

Ingredients:

- 1 pound chicken breasts, cut into bite-sized pieces
- 1 pound bacon, preferably thin-cut for easy wrapping
- Optional: Salt and pepper for seasoning (if you include these in your version of the carnivore diet)

Instructions:

1. Preparation: Preheat your oven to 400°F (200°C). If you prefer to use an air fryer, you'll still follow the same preparation steps but refer to your device's manual for cooking times and temperatures.
2. Wrap the Chicken: Take a piece of chicken breast and wrap it with bacon. Secure with a toothpick if needed. Repeat until all chicken is wrapped. For carnivore dieters, keep seasonings minimal and within guidelines.
3. Cooking: Place the bacon-wrapped chicken bites on a baking sheet lined with parchment paper for easier cleanup. Ensure they're not touching, to allow the bacon to crisp up evenly.
4. Bake: Transfer the baking sheet to the preheated oven. Bake for 25-30 minutes, or until the bacon is crispy and the chicken is thoroughly cooked. The cooking time might vary depending on the thickness of your chicken and bacon, so keep an eye on them.

5. Alternative Cooking Methods: For those using an air fryer, cook the bacon-wrapped chicken bites at 400°F for about 15-20 minutes, or until crispy and fully cooked. You might need to work in batches depending on the size of your air fryer.
6. Serving: Once cooked, remove the bacon chicken bites from the oven or air fryer and let them rest for a few minutes on a plate lined with a paper towel to absorb any excess fat.
7. Enjoy: Serve your Carnivore Diet-Friendly Bacon Chicken Bites hot as a delicious and satisfying appetizer or snack. They're perfect for enjoying any time you need a high-protein, zero-carb treat.

Baked Chicken Breast

Ingredients:

- 2 large chicken breasts (boneless and skinless)
- Salt (optional, depending on your dietary approach within the carnivore diet)
- Animal fat (such as tallow or ghee) for greasing

Instructions:

1. Preheat Oven: Start by preheating your oven to 375°F (190°C). This temperature ensures that the chicken cooks through evenly without drying out.
2. Prepare the Chicken: If you're including salt in your version of the carnivore diet, lightly season both sides of the chicken breasts with salt. This step is optional and can be skipped if you prefer not to include any seasoning.
3. Grease the Baking Dish: Use a small amount of animal fat (tallow or ghee) to grease the bottom of a baking dish. This will prevent the chicken from sticking and add an extra layer of flavor.
4. Bake the Chicken: Place chicken breasts in a greased baking dish, ensuring they are spaced apart. Bake in preheated oven for 20-30 minutes, adjusting based on thickness. Use a meat thermometer to ensure internal temp reaches 165°F (74°C) for thorough cooking.

5. Rest Before Serving: Once the chicken is fully cooked, remove it from the oven and let it rest for a few minutes. This allows the juices to redistribute throughout the meat, ensuring that each bite is moist and flavorful.
6. Serve and Enjoy: Serve the baked chicken breast as is for a carnivore meal. To boost enjoyment and stick to the diet, pair it with other animal-based foods like fried eggs or cheese, if dairy fits your approach.

Beef and Liver Burger

Ingredients:

- 1 pound ground beef (preferably grass-fed for higher nutrient content)
- 1/2 pound beef liver, finely chopped or ground
- Salt (optional, to taste, based on your dietary preferences within the carnivore diet)
- Animal fat (such as tallow or ghee) for cooking

Instructions:

1. Prepare the Meat Mixture: In a large bowl, combine the ground beef and finely chopped or ground beef liver. If you're including salt in your version of the carnivore diet, add it to the mixture according to your taste preference. Mix well until the beef and liver are thoroughly combined.
2. Form the Patties: Divide the meat mixture into equal portions, shaping each into a burger patty. The size and thickness of the patties can be adjusted based on personal preference, but ensure they're uniform for even cooking.
3. Preheat Your Cooking Surface: Heat a skillet or grill over medium-high heat. Add a small amount of animal fat (tallow or ghee) to grease the surface and prevent sticking. If using a grill, ensure the grates are well-greased.

4. Cook the Burgers: Place the patties on the hot skillet or grill. Cook for about 3-5 minutes on each side, or until the desired level of doneness is achieved. The cooking time will vary depending on the thickness of the patties and how well done you prefer your burgers.
5. Rest Before Serving: Once cooked, transfer the burgers to a plate and let them rest for a few minutes. This allows the juices to settle, ensuring your burgers will be moist and flavorful.
6. Serve and Enjoy: Serve your Beef and Liver Burgers as is for a pure carnivore meal. For those who include dairy in their carnivore diet, topping the burger with a slice of cheese could add an extra layer of flavor.

Healthy Beef Brisket

Ingredients:

- 3-4 pounds of beef brisket (choose a cut with a good amount of fat for the best flavor and tenderness)
- Salt (optional, depending on your personal dietary preferences within the carnivore diet framework)

Instructions:

1. Preheat Your Oven: Begin by setting your oven to a low temperature of 275°F (135°C). The slow cooking process is key to making the brisket tender and flavorful.
2. Prepare the Brisket: If you're opting to use salt, season the brisket generously on all sides. While the carnivore diet primarily focuses on animal products, the addition of salt can enhance the natural flavors of the meat.
3. Ready the Pan: Place your brisket in a large roasting pan. Choosing a pan with enough space ensures the brisket cooks evenly. There's no need to add liquids or cover the brisket, as its own fat will keep it moist during the cooking process.
4. Bake Slowly: Transfer the pan to the preheated oven. The brisket will need to be baked for approximately 6 hours. This long cooking time allows the tough fibers in the brisket to break down, resulting in incredibly tender meat.

5. Check for Doneness: The brisket is done when it's tender enough to be easily pierced with a fork. If you find the brisket isn't quite there yet, don't hesitate to give it more time in the oven. Patience is key!
6. Rest Before Slicing: Once removed from the oven, let the brisket rest for about 20-30 minutes. This resting period allows the juices to redistribute throughout the meat, ensuring it's moist and flavorful when sliced.
7. Slice Against the Grain: When you're ready to serve, slice the brisket against the grain. This means cutting perpendicular to the muscle fibers, which makes the slices more tender and enjoyable to eat.
8. Serve and Enjoy: Serve your healthy beef brisket as the centerpiece of your meal. It needs no accompaniment to shine on the carnivore diet, offering deep, satisfying flavors and a wealth of nutrients.

Beef Heart

Ingredients:

- 1 beef heart (approximately 2-3 lbs), trimmed and cut into 1-inch cubes
- Salt (optional, depending on personal preference)

Instructions:

1. Prepare the Beef Heart: Rinse the beef heart under cold water, pat dry with paper towels, and trim off any fat and silver skin. Cut into 1-inch cubes for even cooking.
2. Optional Seasoning: Lightly season beef heart cubes with salt if desired for the carnivore diet.

Cooking the Beef Heart:

3. Skillet Method: Sear beef heart cubes in a single layer in a heated skillet for 2-3 minutes on each side. Remove and let rest.
4. Oven Method: Roast beef heart cubes on a baking sheet at 375°F for 10-15 minutes for desired doneness.

Blackened Shrimp

Ingredients:

- 1 pound large shrimp, peeled and deveined
- Animal fat (such as tallow, ghee, or butter), for cooking
- Salt (optional, depending on personal preference)

Instructions:

1. Prepare the Shrimp: Clean, peel, and devein the shrimp. Pat dry with paper towels to remove excess moisture for a good sear.
2. Heat the Cooking Fat: In a large skillet over medium-high heat, melt your chosen animal fat (tallow, ghee, or butter) until hot. Ensure the fat is thin but completely covers the skillet bottom.
3. Optional Seasoning: If salt is part of your carnivore diet, lightly season the shrimp with salt. This step is flexible based on your dietary preferences.
4. Cook the Shrimp: Add shrimp in a single layer to the hot, shimmering fat. Cook for about 2 minutes until pink and slightly charred.
5. Flip and Finish Cooking: Flip the shrimp and cook for 1-2 minutes until fully pink and opaque. Cooking time varies with shrimp size.

6. Serve Immediately: Transfer blackened shrimp to a plate and serve right away. The shrimp should be juicy inside with a slightly crispy exterior.
7. Optional Serving Suggestions: While delicious on their own, those including dairy in their carnivore diet can enjoy the shrimp with melted butter or ghee for dipping.

Chicken Enchilada

Ingredients:

- 2 pounds chicken breasts, cooked and shredded
- 8 ounces cream cheese (ensure it's pure cream cheese, with no added non-carnivore ingredients)
- 2 cups shredded cheddar cheese, divided
- 1 cup sour cream
- Salt (optional, according to taste)

Instructions:

1. Preheat Oven: Preheat your oven to 350°F (175°C) while preparing enchilada filling.
2. Prepare Chicken Filling: Mix cooked, shredded chicken with cream cheese, 1 cup of cheddar cheese, and sour cream. Add salt to taste if desired.
3. Form "Enchiladas": Spoon chicken mixture onto a baking dish, shaping into cylinders.
4. Add Cheese Topping: Sprinkle remaining cheddar cheese over enchiladas.
5. Bake: Bake for 20-25 minutes until cheese is melted and golden.
6. Serve: Let cool before enjoying these delicious carnivore diet-friendly chicken enchiladas.

Crispy Chicken Thighs

Ingredients:

- 4 chicken thighs (with skin on for maximum crispiness)
- Salt (optional, based on your dietary preferences within the carnivore diet)
- Animal fat (such as tallow, ghee, or duck fat) for greasing the pan, if needed

Instructions:

1. Preheat Oven: Preheat to 400°F (200°C) for crispy skin.
2. Prepare Chicken: Pat dry chicken thighs, and season with salt.
3. Grease Pan (If Needed): Lightly grease the pan if the thighs are lean.
4. Arrange Chicken: Place skin-side up on the pan.
5. Bake: Bake for 35-45 minutes until golden and crispy.
6. Check Doneness: Juices clear, internal temp 165°F (74°C).
7. Serve: Rest cooked thighs before serving.

Crockpot Shredded Chicken

Ingredients:

- 2-3 pounds of boneless, skinless chicken breasts or thighs
- Salt (optional, based on your dietary preferences)
- Water or homemade animal-based broth (if desired, for added moisture, though not necessary)

Instructions:

1. Prepare the Chicken: Lightly season the chicken with salt if it's part of your carnivore diet. Adjust based on your preferences.
2. Arrange in the Crockpot: Place the chicken in the crockpot. For more moist shredded chicken, add a bit of water or homemade animal-based broth. The chicken will release juices as it cooks.
3. Cooking Time: Cover and cook on low for 6-8 hours or on high for 3-4 hours until tender for easy shredding.
4. Shred the Chicken: Use two forks to shred the fully cooked chicken in the crockpot. Remove excess liquid if needed.
5. Serve or Store: Enjoy immediately or refrigerate for later use. Use it as is or as a base for other carnivore diet dishes.

6. Optional Serving Suggestions: For added richness, mix in melted butter or ghee with the shredded chicken, especially if dairy is part of your carnivore diet.

Grilled Chicken Kebabs

Ingredients:

- 2 pounds chicken breast or thigh meat, cut into 1½-inch pieces
- Salt (optional, depending on your dietary preferences)
- Animal fat (such as tallow, ghee, or butter), melted, for brushing

Instructions:

1. Preheat the Grill: Get your grill to medium-high heat, around 375°F to 400°F (190°C to 204°C), for perfectly cooked chicken with a nice char.
2. Prepare the Chicken: Lightly season the chicken with salt if desired for the carnivore diet.
3. Thread the Chicken: Skewer the chicken pieces, ensuring even spacing for thorough cooking.
4. Brush with Fat: Coat the chicken with melted animal fat to prevent sticking and add flavor.
5. Grill the Kebabs: Grill the skewers for 10-15 minutes, turning regularly until charred and cooked through.
6. Rest Before Serving: Let the cooked skewers rest briefly to enhance tenderness and flavor.
7. Serve and Enjoy: Your Grilled Chicken Kebabs are ready to be savored, highlighting the natural flavors with a touch of grilling and optional salt.

Grilled Flank Steak

Ingredients:

- 1.5 to 2 pounds flank steak
- Salt (optional, based on your dietary preferences)

Instructions:

1. Prepare the Grill: Preheat the grill to high heat for a nice sear on the steak, locking in natural juices.
2. Prepare the Flank Steak: Season both sides liberally with salt if desired in your carnivore diet.
3. Grill the Steak: Cook flank steak for 5-7 minutes each side for medium-rare. Adjust time for preferred doneness; internal temp should reach 130°F (54°C).
4. Rest the Steak: Let the steak rest on a cutting board for 5-10 minutes to redistribute juices for juiciness and flavor.
5. Slice and Serve: Slice steak thinly against the grain for tenderness.
6. Enjoy: Serve immediately for a satisfying, nutrient-dense meal on the carnivore diet.

Italian Burgers

Ingredients:

- 2 pounds ground beef (choose a higher fat content for juicier burgers)
- 1/2 cup grated Parmesan cheese (ensure it's pure Parmesan with no fillers)
- 1 tablespoon rendered animal fat (beef tallow or pork lard) for cooking
- Salt (optional, depending on your dietary preferences)
- 1 teaspoon ground black pepper (optional and only if you include spices in your version of the carnivore diet)

Instructions:

1. Prep the Grill or Skillet: Preheat your grill to high heat or heat a skillet over medium-high heat on the stove. If using a skillet, add the rendered animal fat to grease the pan lightly.
2. Mix the Burger Patties: In a big bowl, mix ground beef, Parmesan, salt, and pepper. Gently combine. Avoid overworking the meat to keep burgers juicy.
3. Form the Patties: Divide the mixture into 6 equal portions (or adjust for your patty size). Shape each into a patty, creating a slight indentation in the center with your thumb for even cooking.

4. Cook the Burgers: Place the patties on the grill or in the skillet. Cook for about 4 minutes per side for medium-rare burgers. Adjust time based on your preference. Use a meat thermometer to check for doneness; aim for 130°F (54°C) for medium-rare.
5. Rest the Burgers: time-basedOnce cooked to your liking, transfer the burgers to a plate and let them rest for a few minutes. This allows the juices to redistribute, enhancing flavor and moisture.
6. Serve and Enjoy: Serve the Italian Burgers hot. On the carnivore diet, enjoy them alone or with animal-based products like whipped cream or butter to enhance the meal's richness.

Lamb Chops

Ingredients:

- 4 lamb chops (about 1 inch thick)
- Salt (optional, based on your dietary preferences)
- 2 tablespoons rendered animal fat (such as tallow or lard) for cooking if needed

Instructions:

1. Preheat Cooking Surface: If grilling, preheat to high heat. For pan-searing, use a heavy skillet (cast iron works well) over medium-high heat. If lamb chops are lean, add rendered animal fat to prevent sticking and ensure even cooking.
2. Prepare the Lamb Chops: When following the carnivore diet, season lamb chops with salt to taste on both sides. This step is optional and can be adjusted based on your dietary preferences.
3. Cook the Lamb Chops: Once the cooking surface is hot, add the lamb chops to the grill or skillet. For medium-rare, cook each side for 3-4 minutes, adjusting based on thickness and preferred doneness. Use a meat thermometer; at 145°F (63°C) for medium-rare.
4. Rest the Lamb Chops: After cooking, move the lamb chops to a plate and let them rest for 5 minutes. Resting redistributes juices in the meat, making every bite juicy and flavorful.

5. Serve and Enjoy: After resting, serve the lamb chops promptly. Enjoy them as they are, highlighting the succulent lamb flavors. For dairy-inclusive carnivores, try adding butter or ghee on top for extra richness.

Lime Coconut Skirt Steak

Ingredients:

- 2 pounds skirt steak
- Salt (optional, to taste)
- Animal fat (for cooking, if needed)

Instructions:

1. Preparation: If using salt, generously season both sides of the skirt steak. Adjust salt amount based on preference and dietary guidelines.
2. Preheat the Grill or Pan: Preheat your grill to high heat or a cast-iron skillet to high heat. If using a skillet and your steak is very lean, consider adding a bit of animal fat (like tallow or lard) to prevent sticking and ensure an even sear.
3. Cook the Steak: Place the skirt steak on the grill or skillet. Cook 3-4 minutes per side for medium-rare, adjusting based on preferred doneness. Skirt steak stays tender with a hot, quick cook.
4. Rest the Steak: After cooking, move the steak to a cutting board and let it rest for 5 minutes. Resting helps juices spread in the meat for a tastier, juicier steak.

5. Serve: Slice the steak against the grain into thin strips. This is crucial for skirt steak, as it helps break up the muscle fibers and makes the meat more tender and easier to chew.

Moroccan Kouah

Ingredients:

- 1 pound mixed lamb heart and kidney, bite-sized pieces
- Salt (optional)
- Animal fat (tallow or lard) for grilling

Instructions:

1. Preparation: Clean the lamb's heart and kidney. Remove excess fat or connective tissue from the heart, soak the kidney in cold water to remove bitterness, changing water a few times. Pat dry with paper towels.
2. Season (Optional): Lightly season heart and kidney pieces with salt if desired. Adjust according to dietary choices.
3. Skewer the Offal: Thread heart and kidney pieces onto skewers, alternating for flavor and texture. Soak wooden skewers in water for 30 minutes to prevent burning.
4. Preheat the Grill: Preheat the grill to medium-high. Use a cast-iron skillet or grill pan on the stove over medium-high heat if grilling isn't possible. Add animal fat to prevent sticking.
5. Grill the Kouah: Grill skewers on each side for 3-4 minutes until cooked through but tender. High heat sears outside quickly, sealing in juices.

6. Serve Immediately: Remove Kouah from heat once grilled. Let rest for a couple of minutes before serving to redistribute juices.
7. Enjoy: Serve hot, right off the grill or skillet. Emphasizes offal's natural flavors, aligning with the carnivore diet's focus on animal-based nutrition.

Pork Tenderloin

Ingredients:

- 1 pork tenderloin (approximately 1 to 1.5 pounds)
- Salt (optional, according to your dietary preferences)
- Animal fat (such as lard or tallow), if needed for cooking

Instructions:

1. Preheat Your Oven: Begin by preheating your oven to 375°F (190°C). This moderate temperature will cook the pork tenderloin through without drying it out.
2. Prepare the Pork Tenderloin: If you're including salt in your diet, season the pork tenderloin lightly with salt all over. This step is optional and can be adjusted based on personal dietary choices.
3. Sear the Tenderloin: Heat a skillet or oven-proof pan over medium-high heat. If the tenderloin is lean, add a little animal fat to prevent sticking and achieve a nice sear. Sear the pork tenderloin on all sides until golden brown, about 2-3 minutes per side.
4. Roast the Tenderloin: Transfer the skillet with the pork into the preheated oven. Roast for 15-20 minutes until the pork reaches 145°F (63°C) internally. Cooking time varies based on size and thickness, so use a meat thermometer for accuracy.

5. Rest Before Serving: Once cooked, take the pork tenderloin out of the oven and let it rest for at least 5 minutes before slicing. Resting redistributes juices in the meat for moist, flavorful slices.
6. Serve and Enjoy: Slice the pork tenderloin into medallions and serve immediately. As a dish following the carnivore diet guidelines, it stands alone beautifully without the need for additional accompaniments.

Prosciutto-Roast Beef Tenderloin

Ingredients:

- 1 whole beef tenderloin (approximately 2-3 pounds)
- 10-12 slices of prosciutto
- Salt (optional, to taste)

Instructions:

1. Prepare the Beef Tenderloin: Start by preparing your beef tenderloin. If you prefer, lightly season the tenderloin with salt. This is optional and can be adjusted based on personal dietary preferences.
2. Wrap with Prosciutto: Arrange prosciutto slices on a flat surface, slightly overlapping to form a sheet. Wrap the beef tenderloin in the prosciutto, ensuring full coverage. The prosciutto fat enhances moisture and flavor during cooking.
3. Preheat the Oven: Preheat your oven to 400°F (200°C). A hot oven will ensure a nicely browned exterior while keeping the inside tender and juicy.
4. Roast the Tenderloin: Place the tenderloin on a rack in a roasting pan for air circulation. Roast in the oven for 25-30 minutes for medium-rare, or until it reaches your preferred doneness. Use a meat thermometer to check for 135°F (57°C) for medium-rare.
5. Rest Before Serving: After cooking, take the tenderloin out of the oven and let it rest for at least 10 minutes

before slicing. Resting helps the juices spread evenly in the meat, keeping every slice flavorful and moist.
6. Serve: Slice the tenderloin into medallions and serve immediately. Enjoy the rich flavors of the beef complemented by the savory prosciutto.

Roasted Chicken

Ingredients:

- 1 whole chicken (about 4 to 5 pounds)
- Salt (optional, to taste)
- Animal fat (such as duck fat, lard, or tallow), if needed for extra juiciness

Instructions:

1. Preheat Your Oven: Begin by preheating your oven to 425°F (220°C). This high temperature will help to crisp the skin while keeping the inside juicy.
2. Prepare the Chicken: Season inside and outside of the chicken with salt. This step is optional and can be adjusted based on personal preferences. For lean chicken, add fat for flavor and moistness by rubbing a small amount of animal fat on the outside.
3. Truss the Chicken (Optional): For even cooking and to maintain the chicken's shape while roasting, tie its legs together with twine and tuck the wing tips under the body. This step is optional.
4. Roast the Chicken: Place the chicken breast side up in a roasting pan or on a rack in the oven. Roast for about 1 hour and 15 minutes until juices run clear when cutting between leg and thigh, and thigh reaches 165°F (74°C).

5. Rest Before Serving: After cooking the chicken, take it out of the oven and let it rest for at least 10 minutes before cutting. Resting helps distribute the juices evenly, making each bite flavorful and juicy.
6. Serve: Carve the chicken into pieces and serve immediately. Enjoy the succulent flavors of the roasted chicken as a fulfilling main course.

Salmon Filet with Garlic and Pepper

Ingredients:

- 2 salmon filets (6-8 ounces each)
- Salt (optional, to taste)

Instructions:

1. Preheat the Grill or Pan: If using a grill, preheat to medium-high. For pan-searing, heat a skillet over medium-high on the stove. Skin-on salmon filets with natural fat may not need extra fat. Lean cuts or skinless filets might benefit from a bit of animal fat (tallow or lard) to prevent sticking and boost flavor.
2. Prepare the Salmon: If including salt in your diet, lightly season the salmon filets with salt on both sides. This step is optional and based on personal dietary preferences.
3. Cook the Salmon: Place salmon filets on a grill or in a skillet. If skin-on, start with skin down. Cook for 4-5 minutes on the first side, then flip and cook 3-4 minutes more, or until salmon is cooked to your liking. Cooking time varies with filet thickness.
4. Serve Immediately: Once cooked to your preference, remove the salmon filets from the heat and serve immediately.

Salmon Wrapped in Bacon

Ingredients:

- 4 salmon fillets (6-8 ounces each)
- 8-12 slices of bacon (2-3 slices per salmon fillet, depending on size)

Instructions:

1. Prepare the Salmon and Bacon: Preheat the oven to 400°F (200°C) for oven baking. Or, use a skillet on the stove for a crispier finish. Pat the salmon fillets dry with paper towels to help the bacon stick better.
2. Wrap the Salmon: Lay 2-3 bacon slices slightly overlapping. Roll a salmon fillet tightly in the bacon, covering as much salmon as possible. Repeat for all fillets. Secure bacon with toothpicks if needed during cooking.

Oven Baking Method:

3. Place bacon-wrapped salmon fillets on a wire rack on a baking sheet to cook evenly and crisp up the bacon.
4. Bake in the preheated oven for 15-20 minutes until the bacon is crispy and the salmon is cooked through, timing varies based on fillet thickness and bacon preference.

Stovetop Method:

5. Heat a large skillet over medium-high heat. Add the bacon-wrapped salmon fillets seam-side down to seal the bacon around the salmon.
6. Cook for 3-4 minutes on each side until the bacon is crispy and the salmon is cooked through. Adjust the heat as needed to prevent burning the bacon while ensuring the salmon is fully cooked.
7. Rest and Serve: Once cooked, remove the salmon from the oven or skillet and let it rest for a few minutes before serving. This allows the juices to be redistributed, making the salmon moist and flavorful.
8. Enjoy: Serve the Bacon-Wrapped Salmon right away to enjoy the mix of soft, flaky salmon and crispy, savory bacon. No need for extra seasonings or sides, fitting perfectly in the carnivore diet.

Steaks with Olive Oil

Ingredients:

- 2 steaks (ribeye, sirloin, or your choice of cut), approximately 1-inch thick
- Salt (optional, to taste)
- Animal fat (such as tallow, lard, or butter) for cooking

Instructions:

1. Prepare the Steaks: Allow the steaks to come to room temperature by taking them out of the refrigerator about 30 minutes before you plan to cook them. This helps in cooking the steaks evenly. If you're incorporating salt into your carnivore diet, you can season the steaks lightly on both sides.
2. Preheat Your Cooking Surface: Preheat a skillet, preferably cast iron for its even heat distribution and ability to become very hot, over medium-high to high heat. You want the skillet extremely hot to ensure a good sear on the steaks.
3. Add Fat to Skillet: Add a generous amount of animal fat (tallow, lard, or butter) to the skillet. Allow it to melt and get hot, but not smoking.
4. Cook the Steaks: Once the skillet and fat are hot, add the steaks. Cook without moving for 3-4 minutes on one side based on thickness. Flip and cook 3-4 minutes more for medium-rare. Optionally baste steaks with

pan fat for extra flavor. Adjust times to your preference.
5. Rest the Steaks: After cooking, transfer the steaks to a plate and let them rest for about 5 minutes. Resting allows the juices to redistribute throughout the meat, ensuring that each bite is juicy and flavorful.
6. Serve: Serve the steaks immediately after resting. Enjoy the rich, unadulterated flavors of the meat, enhanced by the natural cooking fats.

Conclusion

Congratulations on completing this guide on the Carnivore Diet for Managing Depression! By now, you've taken a significant step toward understanding how dietary choices can influence mental health and well-being. Embracing the carnivore diet as a potential tool to combat depression is a bold move, reflecting your commitment to exploring all avenues for improving your mental health.

Remember, the journey you're embarking on is deeply personal and unique to your body's needs and responses. The insights you've gained here about the potential benefits of consuming primarily animal products—ranging from reduced inflammation to stabilized blood sugar levels and enhanced nutrient absorption—serve as a foundation for experimenting with the carnivore diet in a way that feels right for you.

It's important to approach this dietary shift with an open mind and a spirit of curiosity. Listen to your body and be willing to adjust as necessary. Finding the right balance might take time, and that's perfectly okay. Every step you take is a step toward discovering what works best for you and your mental health.

Be encouraged by the stories of others who have found relief from depression through dietary changes, but also stay grounded in your own experience. Your health journey is as individual as you are, and what works for one person may not work for another.

As you move forward, don't hesitate to seek support from healthcare professionals, nutritionists, and communities who share your interest in the carnivore diet. Their guidance and experience can be invaluable as you navigate the nuances of this dietary approach.

In closing, give yourself a hearty pat on the back for completing this guide and for your willingness to explore the carnivore diet as a means to manage depression. Your proactive stance on mental health is commendable, and your journey is just beginning. Here's to finding balance, wellness, and joy on your path ahead.

FAQ

Can the carnivore diet help manage depression?

Yes, many individuals report improvements in mood and a reduction in depression symptoms when following a carnivore diet. This might be attributed to the elimination of potentially side-inflammatory foods and an increase in nutrient-dense, mood-enhancing animal products.

What foods are included in the carnivore diet?

The carnivore diet consists exclusively of animal products, including meat, fish, eggs, and certain dairy products. It excludes all plant-based foods.

How quickly can I see results in my mood after starting the carnivore diet?

While individual experiences vary, some report feeling improvements in their mood and overall well-being within a few weeks of adopting the diet.

Is it safe to follow the carnivore diet long-term?

Opinions on the long-term safety of the carnivore diet differ. It's important to consult with a healthcare professional before making any significant dietary changes, especially for managing conditions like depression.

Will I miss out on essential nutrients by not eating plants?

Animal products can provide the most essential nutrients, but it's crucial to consume a variety of animal foods to cover all nutritional bases. Consider supplementing or periodically reviewing your nutrient status with a healthcare provider.

Can the carnivore diet worsen depression for some people?

As with any diet, individual responses can vary. If you notice a worsening of depression symptoms, it's important to consult with a healthcare professional and reconsider if this dietary approach is right for you.

How do I start the carnivore diet for managing depression?

Begin by gradually eliminating plant-based foods from your diet and increasing your intake of high-quality animal products. Pay close attention to how your body and mood respond to these changes.

References and Helpful Links

Aurelius, C. (2020, December 11). Carnivore diet: Everything you need to know (Updated 2020). Carnivore Aurelius. https://carnivoreaurelius.com/carnivore-diet/

Carnivore diet for women. (n.d.). Google Books. https://books.google.com.ph/books?id=6bPnDwAAQBAJ&pg=PA20-IA7&lpg=PA20-IA7&dq=Stock,+Kevin.+%E2%80%9CSymptoms+and+Cures+when+Starting+the+Carnivore+Diet.%E2%80%9D+Meat+Health,+https://meat.health/knowledge-base/carnivore-diet-symptoms-+and-cures/.+Accessed+6+Feb.+2020.&source=bl&ots=ObEWqRLNDO&sig=ACfU3U3nUuwEW14CuSIIjmcVTlJ_osKSlw&hl=en&sa=X&ved=2ahUKEwj_m_K_homFAxU_bWwGHdQqA-8Q6AF6BAgPEAM

Carter, N. (2020, March 6). Can carnivore diet improve sex life? Healthy With Nicole. https://healthywithnicole.com/journal/can-carnivore-diet-improve-sex-life/

Constantin, M.-M., Nita, I. E., Olteanu, R., Constantin, T., Bucur, S., Matei, C., & Raducan, A. (2019). Significance and impact of dietary factors on systemic lupus erythematosus pathogenesis. Experimental and Therapeutic Medicine, 17(2), 1085–1090. https://doi.org/10.3892/etm.2018.6986

Contributors, W. E. (n.d.). Sex positions for overweight people. WebMD. Retrieved April 11, 2024, from https://www.webmd.com/sex/sex-positions-for-overweight-people

Dupuis, N., Curatolo, N., Benoist, J., & Auvin, S. (2015). Ketogenic diet exhibits anti‑inflammatory properties. Epilepsia, 56(7). https://doi.org/10.1111/epi.13038

Endometriosis: Symptoms, surgery, treatment, diagnosis, causes, pain. (n.d.). MedicineNet. Retrieved April 11, 2024, from https://www.medicinenet.com/endometriosis/article.htm

Fairweather, D. L., & Rose, N. R. (2004). Women and autoimmune diseases1. Emerging Infectious Diseases, 10(11), 2005–2011. https://doi.org/10.3201/eid1011.040367

Fairweather, D., & Rose, N. R. (2004). Women and autoimmune diseases1. Emerging Infectious Diseases, 10(11), 2005–2011. https://doi.org/10.3201/eid1011.040367

Forsythe, C. E., Phinney, S. D., Fernandez, M. L., Quann, E. E., Wood, R. J., Bibus, D. M., Kraemer, W. J., Feinman, R. D., & Volek, J. S. (2008). Comparison of low fat and low carbohydrate diets on circulating fatty acid composition and markers of inflammation. Lipids, 43(1), 65–77. https://doi.org/10.1007/s11745-007-3132-7

Hamblin, J. (2018, September 1). The Jordan Peterson Meat-Only Diet. The Atlantic. https://www.theatlantic.com/health/archive/2018/08/the-peterson-family-meat-cleanse/567613/

Heys, M., Jiang, C., Schooling, C. M., Zhang, W., Cheng, K. K., Lam, T. H., & Leung, G. M. (2010). Is childhood meat eating associated with better later adulthood cognition in a developing population? European

Journal of Epidemiology, 25(7), 507–516. https://doi.org/10.1007/s10654-010-9466-0

Ho, K.-S., Tan, C. Y. M., Mohd Daud, M. A., & Seow-Choen, F. (2012a). Stopping or reducing dietary fiber intake reduces constipation and its associated symptoms. World Journal of Gastroenterology : WJG, 18(33), 4593–4596. https://doi.org/10.3748/wjg.v18.i33.4593

Ho, K.-S., Tan, C. Y. M., Mohd Daud, M. A., & Seow-Choen, F. (2012b). Stopping or reducing dietary fiber intake reduces constipation and its associated symptoms. World Journal of Gastroenterology : WJG, 18(33), 4593–4596. https://doi.org/10.3748/wjg.v18.i33.4593

Hokage, A. (2022, February 1). AIP Diet: Part 14 - The Anonymous Hokage - Medium. Medium. https://medium.com/@bcopublishing/aip-diet-part-14-50c76269767

Hyson, S. (2023, November 29). The Carnivore Diet: Is Eating ONLY Meat Healthy, or Totally F@#$ing Crazy? Onnit Academy. https://www.onnit.com/academy/the-carnivore-diet/

Jurkiewicz-Przondziono, J., Lemm, M., Kwiatkowska-Pamuła, A., Ziółko, E., & Wójtowicz, M. K. (2017). Influence of diet on the risk of developing endometriosis. Ginekologia Polska, 88(2), 96–102. https://doi.org/10.5603/GP.a2017.0017

Kim, J. Y., & Kang, S. W. (2017). Relationships between dietary intake and cognitive function in healthy korean children and adolescents. Journal of Lifestyle Medicine, 7(1), 10–17. https://doi.org/10.15280/jlm.2017.7.1.10

LaManna, J. C., Salem, N., Puchowicz, M., Erokwu, B., Koppaka, S., Flask, C., & Lee, Z. (2009). Ketones suppress brain glucose consumption. Advances in Experimental Medicine and Biology, 645, 301–306. https://doi.org/10.1007/978-0-387-85998-9_45

Ld, L. S. M. R. (2023, March 13). All you need to know about the carnivore (All-Meat) diet. Healthline. https://www.healthline.com/nutrition/carnivore-diet

Maywald, M., & Rink, L. (2017). Zinc supplementation induces CD4+CD25+Foxp3+ antigen-specific regulatory T cells and suppresses IFN-γ production by upregulation of Foxp3 and KLF-10 and downregulation of IRF-1. European Journal of Nutrition, 56(5), 1859–1869. https://doi.org/10.1007/s00394-016-1228-7

mindbodygreen. (2021, April 13). Should you eat a Meat-Only Diet to lose weight, fight pain & cure Depression? Mindbodygreen. https://www.mindbodygreen.com/articles/what-is-the-carnivore-diet

MS, C. K. (2022, September 20). Everything You Need to Know about the Carnivore Diet and How It Can Affect Your Health. Chris Kresser. https://chriskresser.com/the-carnivore-diet-is-it-really-healthy/

Oh, R., Gilani, B., & Uppaluri, K. R. (2023, August 17). Low-Carbohydrate diet. StatPearls - NCBI Bookshelf. https://www.ncbi.nlm.nih.gov/books/NBK537084/

Oh, R., Gilani, B., & Uppaluri, K. R. (2024). Low-carbohydrate diet. In StatPearls. StatPearls Publishing. http://www.ncbi.nlm.nih.gov/books/NBK537084/

Porpora, M. G., Brunelli, R., Costa, G., Imperiale, L., Krasnowska, E. K., Lundeberg, T., Nofroni, I., Piccioni, M. G., Pittaluga, E., Ticino, A., & Parasassi, T. (2013). A promise in the treatment of endometriosis: An observational cohort study on ovarian endometrioma reduction by n-acetylcysteine. Evidence-Based Complementary and Alternative Medicine : eCAM, 2013, 240702. https://doi.org/10.1155/2013/240702

Rd, J. K. (2023, May 8). What is the carnivore diet? Health. https://www.health.com/carnivore-diet-7486099

Rosenkranz, E., Maywald, M., Hilgers, R.-D., Brieger, A., Clarner, T., Kipp, M., Plümäkers, B., Meyer, S., Schwerdtle, T., & Rink, L. (2016). Induction of regulatory T cells in Th1-/Th17-driven experimental autoimmune encephalomyelitis by zinc administration. The Journal of Nutritional Biochemistry, 29, 116–123. https://doi.org/10.1016/j.jnutbio.2015.11.010

Sørensen, L. B., Søe, M., Halkier, K. H., Stigsby, B., & Astrup, A. (2012a). Effects of increased dietary protein-to-carbohydrate ratios in women with polycystic ovary syndrome. The American Journal of Clinical Nutrition, 95(1), 39–48. https://doi.org/10.3945/ajcn.111.020693

Sørensen, L. B., Søe, M., Halkier, K. H., Stigsby, B., & Astrup, A. (2012b). Effects of increased dietary protein-to-carbohydrate ratios in women with polycystic ovary syndrome. The American Journal of Clinical Nutrition, 95(1), 39–48. https://doi.org/10.3945/ajcn.111.020693

The Carnivore Diet Handbook: Get Lean, Strong, and Feel your best ever on a 100% Animal-Based Diet: Suzanne, K.: 9781983118180: Amazon.com: Books. (n.d.). https://www.amazon.com/Carnivore-Diet-Handbook-Strong-Animal-Based/dp/1983118184

www.ingramcontent.com/pod-product-compliance
Lightning Source LLC
LaVergne TN
LVHW012033060526
838201LV00061B/4578